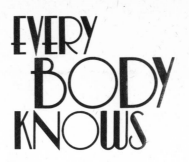

EVERY BODY KNOWS

Yoga demystified

Photographs of Arthur Balaskas,
Mina Balaskas, Kira Balaskas and
Simon Harrison

Photographed by Rosemary Adams

British Broadcasting Corporation

Published to accompany a series of programmes
prepared in consultation with the BBC Further
Education Advisory Council

Published in conjunction with the television
series 'Every Body Knows' first broadcast on
BBC1 on Thursdays at 11.15 pm from
16 January 1975 to 20 March 1975, produced
by Julian Aston, assisted by Ian Rosenbloom

First published 1975
Published by the British Broadcasting
Corporation 35 Marylebone High Street
London W1M 4AA
Printed in England by Billing and Sons Ltd
Guildford, Surrey

ISBN 0 563 10895 9

Introduction

Everybody knows that a great deal of the tension and anxiety that is so much a part of everyday life starts in the mind. However, we rarely connect the physical feelings of stiffness and tension with our mental condition. Of course, mental anxiety need not necessarily have physical repercussions, but the ever-increasing number of people suffering from nervous illnesses does strongly suggest that, in most cases, the body does react very directly to how we are feeling mentally. Until something goes wrong with the body we tend rather to tolerate it, thinking of it often as merely a vehicle with which to transport our heads.

But our bodies are machines of the most intricate and advanced design, capable of a large range of movement, and are potentially highly flexible. Like any machine, the body will only work as well as it is used. Unfortunately the amount of proper use and exercise appears to diminish with each year of life.

Over the last twenty years, an increasing number of people have found that some combination and interpretation of classical physical yoga postures have helped considerably to reduce some of the stress of life. Despite growing popularity, a great deal of mystery still surrounds yoga.

EVERY BODY KNOWS has attempted to demystify yoga, and demonstrate the close connection between physical and mental well-being. Whether body and mind are distinct or part of the same whole is a question best left to philosophers. What we can be reasonably sure about is that, by working with our bodies, we will almost certainly feel better. Nobody would abuse a car or a labour-saving appliance, and expect it to work trouble-free. Yet, much of the time, this is exactly the unrealistic expectation we have of our own bodies.

We hope to have presented the postures in as clear and direct a way as possible. All the movements in this book are, to some extent, within the scope of us all. They are neither for acrobats nor gymnasts. They can be safely practised by anyone, using reasonable common sense. Some will obviously be more difficult than others, and they will all require a degree of conscious effort and concentration at the beginning. Very quickly, as the muscles and joints loosen, the movements will become natural and easy.

Using these postures and balancings as guides, everybody can begin to feel a little less tense, a little more relaxed. There's no mystery in this; yoga postures work directly on the physical repository of stress and tension—our muscles and joints. Yoga works systematically on all parts of the body, helping to relieve tension by stretching and contracting those parts that are most tense—most often the shoulders, neck and hamstrings. A fortnight's daily practice of these movements, taken stage by stage, and as slowly and deliberately as you like, can provide ample proof of the effectiveness of physical yoga.

Before practising the exercises, there are a few simple words of warning

■   There is no competition, no prize. Go as slowly as you like.

■   Feel the stretch, but never strain

■   Stay in each posture as long as is comfortable.

■   Wear loose clothing and, if possible, bathe before and after exercises, although failing to bathe should not be an excuse not to practise.

■   Women, during menstrual periods, are generally advised not to practise any inverted postures.

■   Experiment with postures, and remember to exercise both sides of the body.

■   In order to achieve a balanced programme of exercises each time you practise, try to follow a set of backward bends with a set of forward bends, or vice versa, to avoid stiffness.

■   If you have any history of serious backache or heart trouble, or are undergoing any form of medical treatment, consult your doctor before attempting to practise the postures.

Finally, I hope you enjoy this adventure with your own body as much as I have.

Julian Aston
Producer
EVERY BODY KNOWS

5

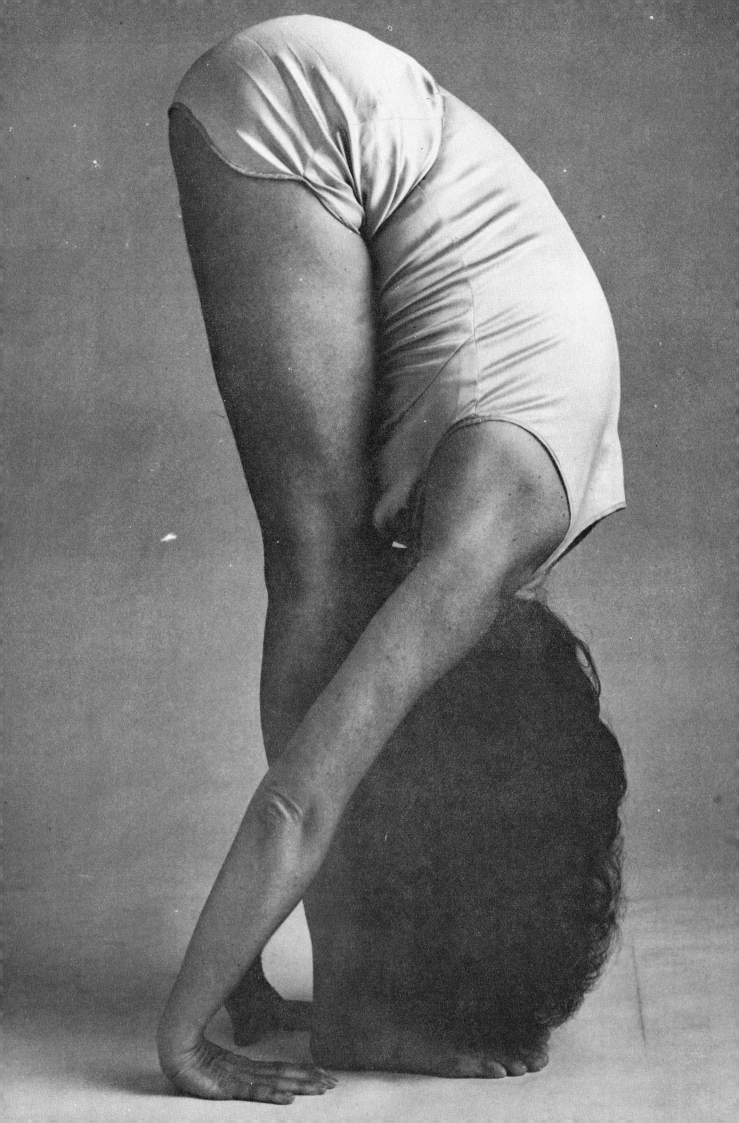

Flexion of pelvis 1

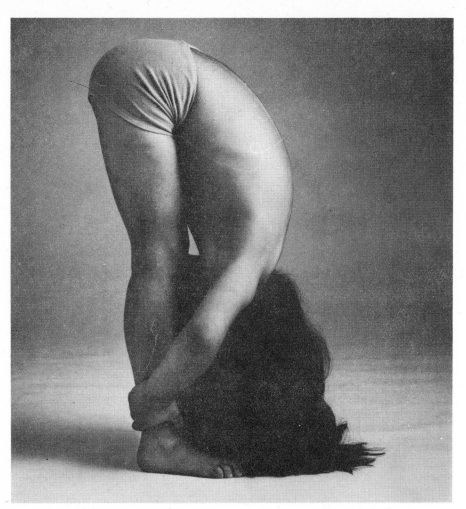

- Start with feet together
(or if easier slightly apart)

- Knees straight

- Allow trunk to go forward, stretching back of thighs and buttocks

- Do not force back but lift buttocks as much as possible

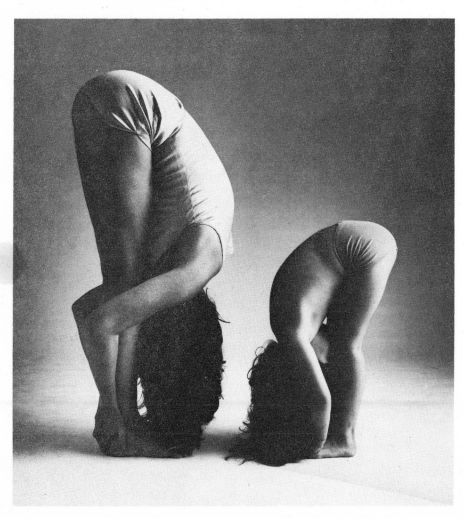

Flexion of pelvis 2

■ Stand with feet five feet apart (five times length of your own foot) and knees straight

■ Heels out, toes in

■ Bend forward from pelvis

■ Buttocks as high as possible

■ Buttocks and back thigh muscles allow the forward bend from hips, not waist

■ Hands on floor at first will assist balance

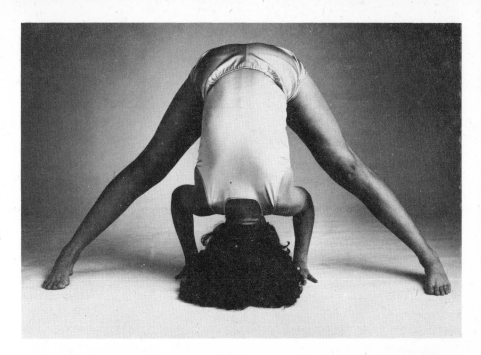

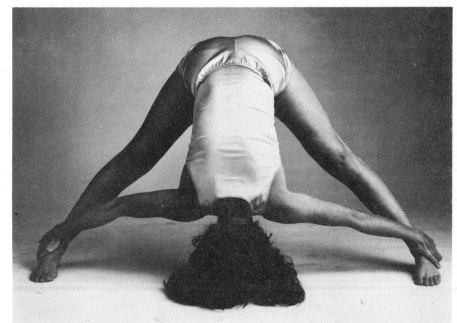

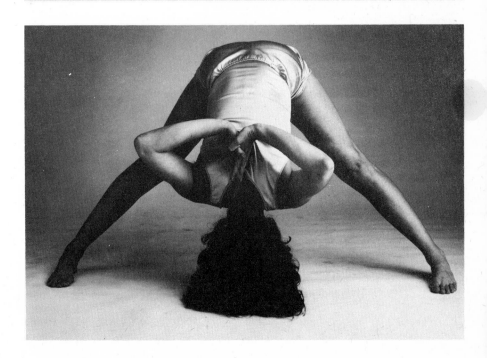

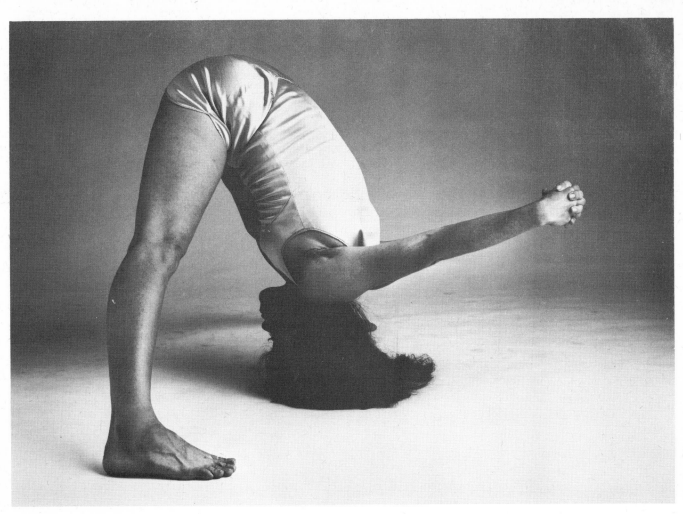

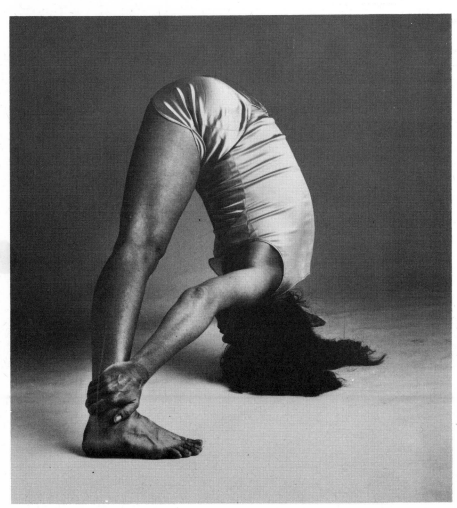

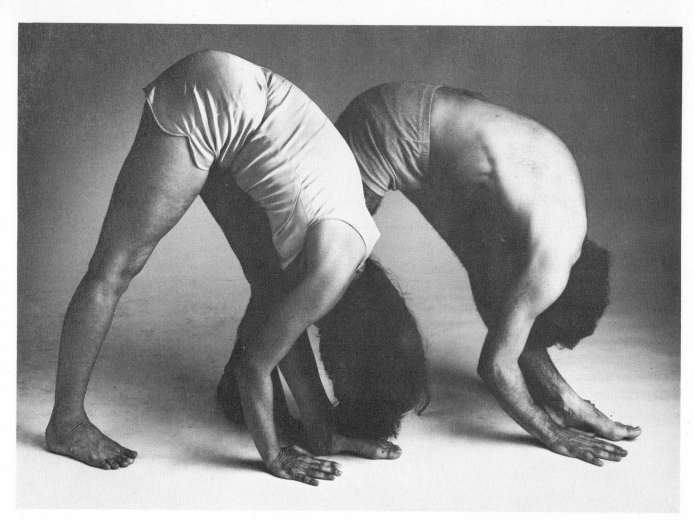

Flexion of pelvis 3

■ From starting position with feet together, move left foot one and a half feet forward, toes pointing straight ahead

■ Move right foot one and a half feet backward, toes turned out at 45°

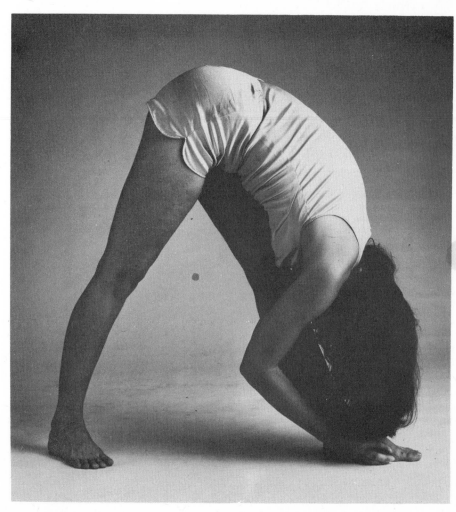

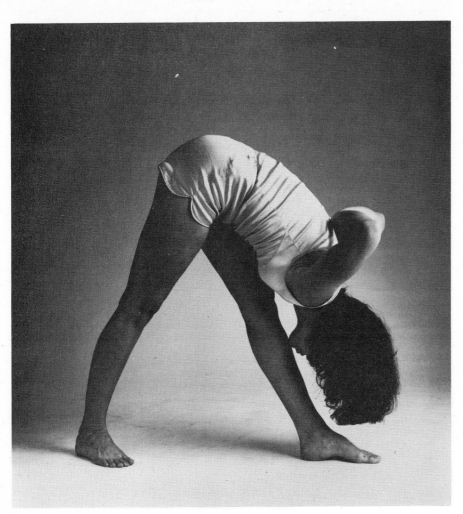

- Allow trunk to go forward from pelvis with little strain on back

- Stretch back of front thigh and buttocks

- Knees straight

- Both feet fully on floor

- Neck and head relaxed

- Repeat starting with right foot

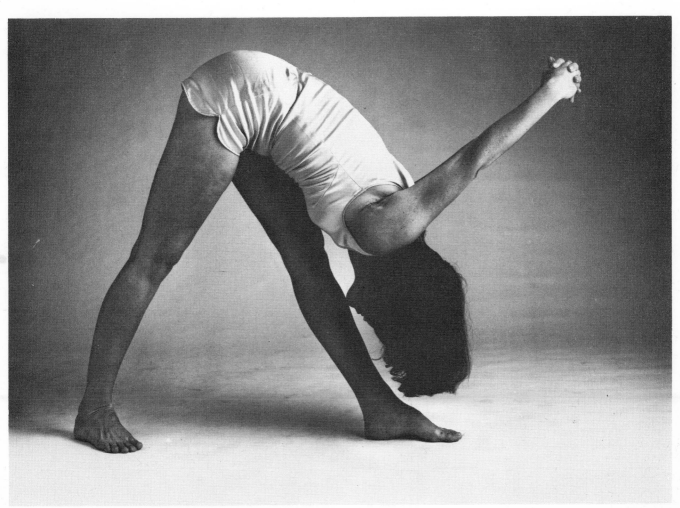

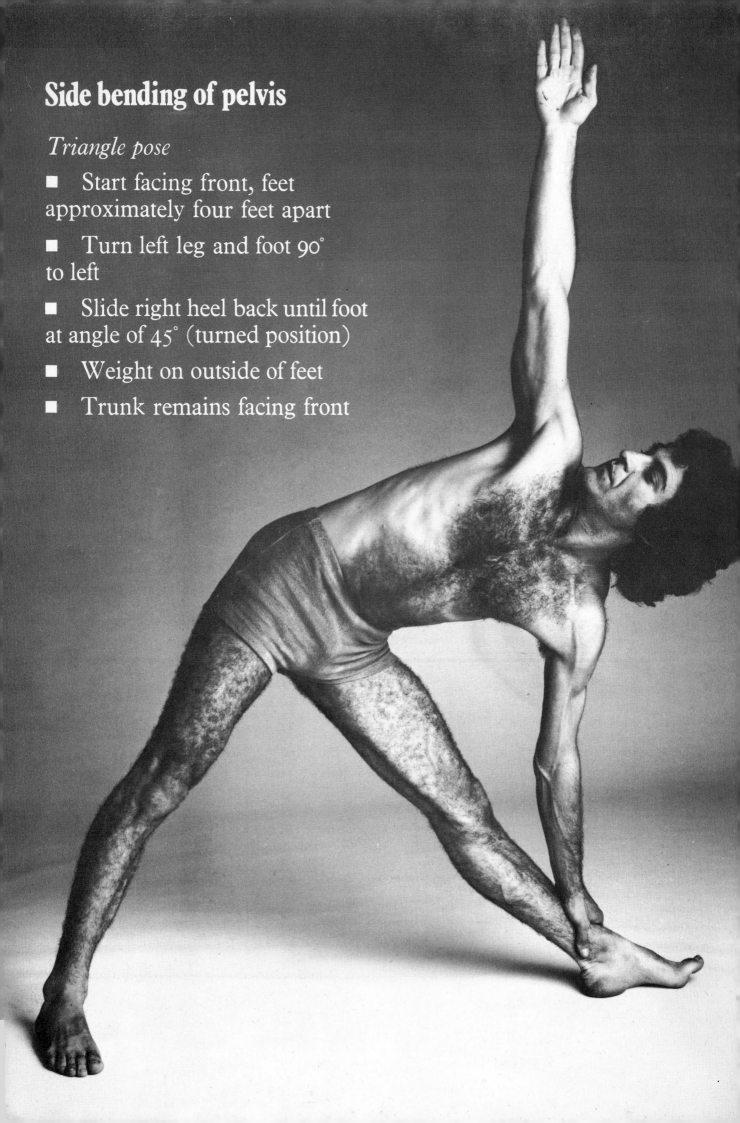

Side bending of pelvis

Triangle pose

- Start facing front, feet approximately four feet apart
- Turn left leg and foot 90° to left
- Slide right heel back until foot at angle of 45° (turned position)
- Weight on outside of feet
- Trunk remains facing front

- Lift arms to shoulder level
- Push right hip to right
- Bend sideways to left
- Turn head to look at right palm
- Aim to touch ankles

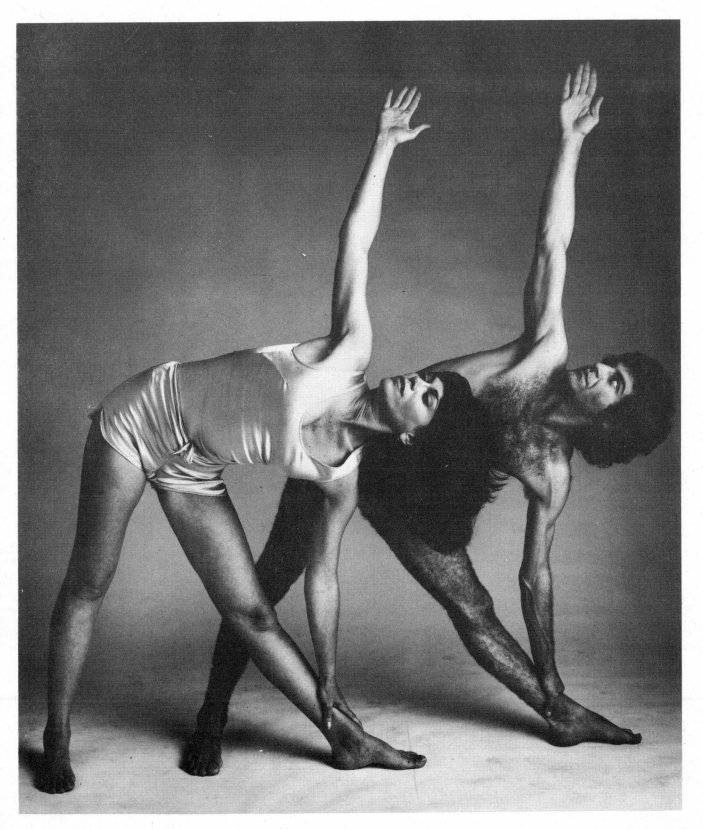

Squatting

- Feet together
- Arms parallel to floor
- Bend knees and squat
- Aim to keep heels on floor (if in difficulty, start with feet slightly apart, and let heels come up)

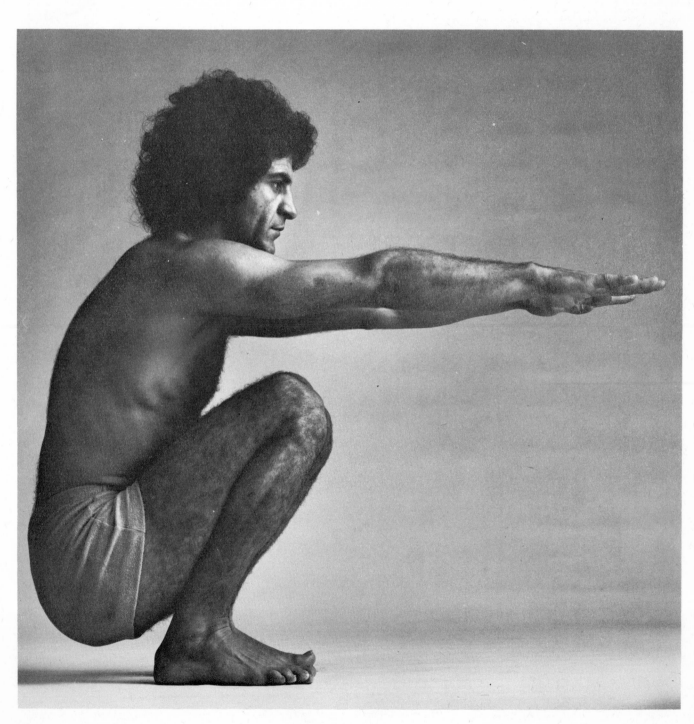

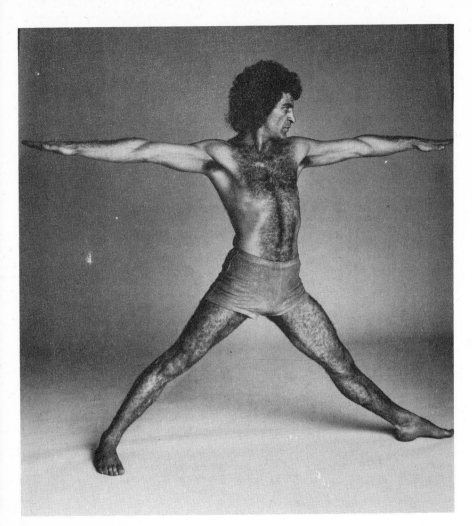

Martial Stance 1

Stage 1

- Feet five feet apart, in turned position, as on page 12
- Feet fully on floor, knees straight
- Arms and hands extended at shoulder level
- Turn trunk from pelvis to face left

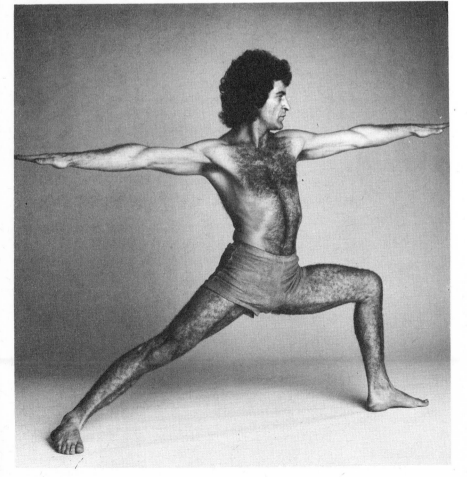

Stage 2

- Bend front knee until thigh parallel to floor
- Shin vertical
- Keep trunk erect
- Try to keep back heel on floor
- Repeat both stages, starting with right foot forward

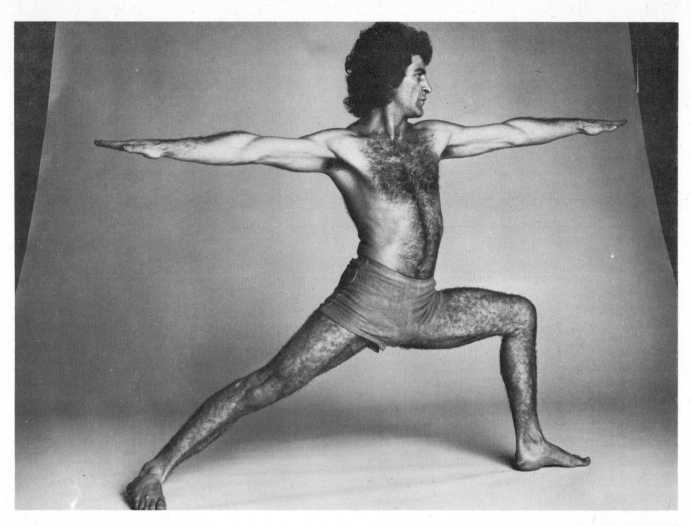

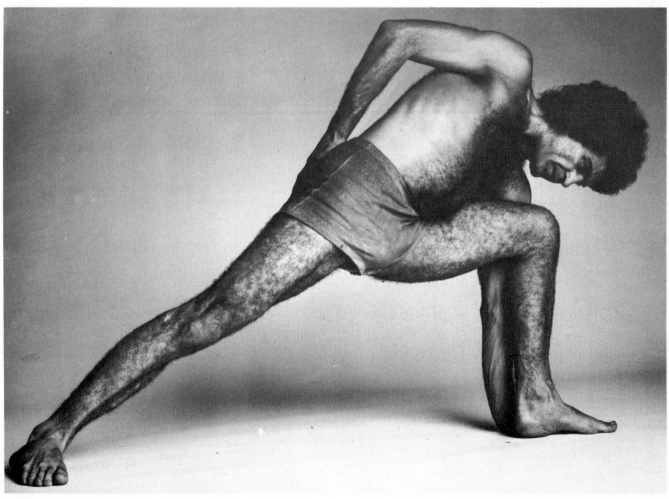

Martial Stance 2

Stage 1

■ Assume Martial Stance 1

Stage 2

■ Lower trunk sideways on to front thigh

■ Palm on floor outside front foot

■ Now roll upper shoulder back and extend other arm over ear

■ Avoid letting pelvis face floor

■ Head turned up

■ Repeat both stages, starting with right leg

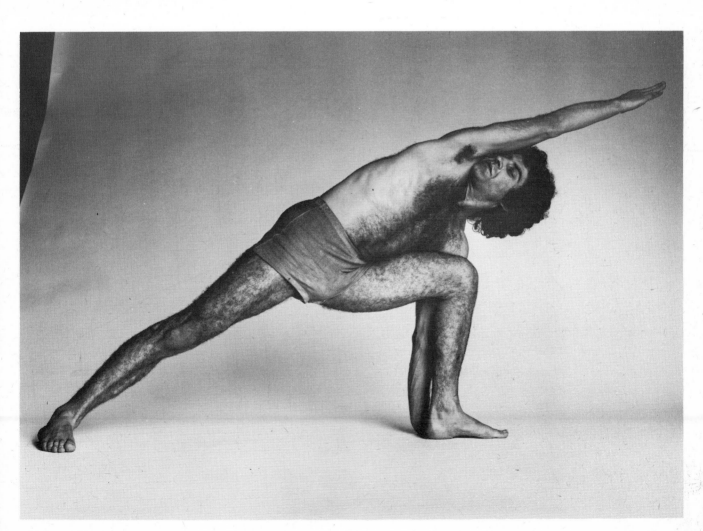

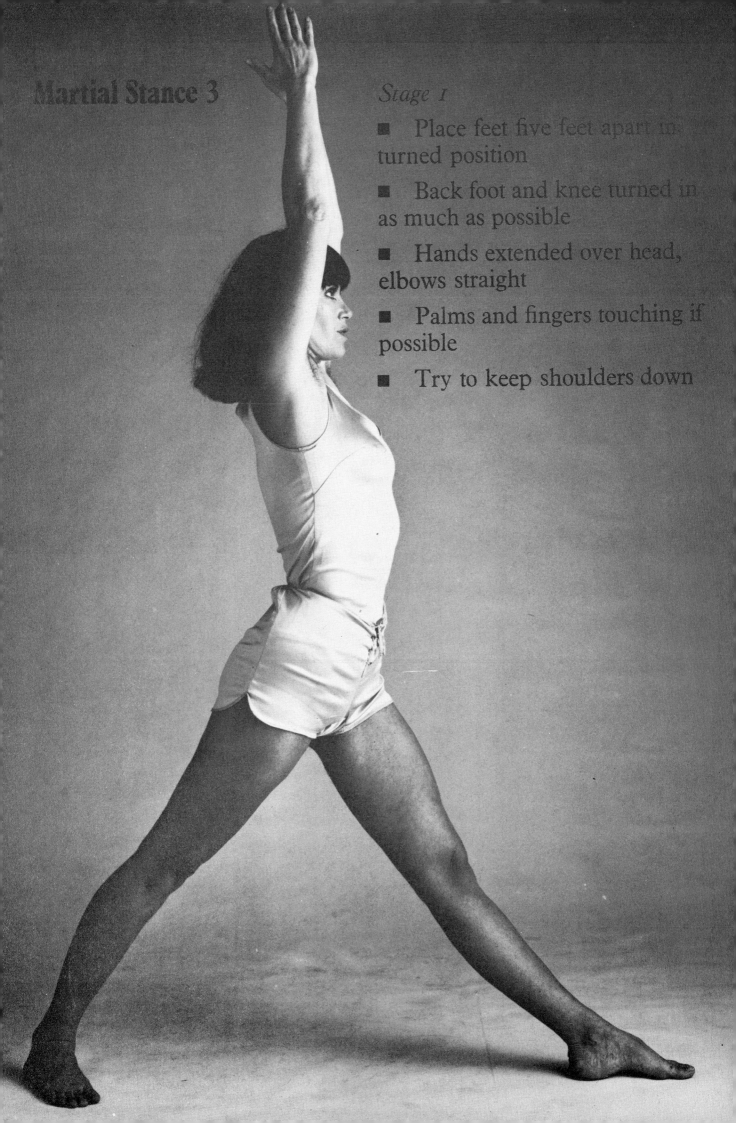

Martial Stance 3

Stage 1

- Place feet five feet apart in turned position
- Back foot and knee turned in as much as possible
- Hands extended over head, elbows straight
- Palms and fingers touching if possible
- Try to keep shoulders down

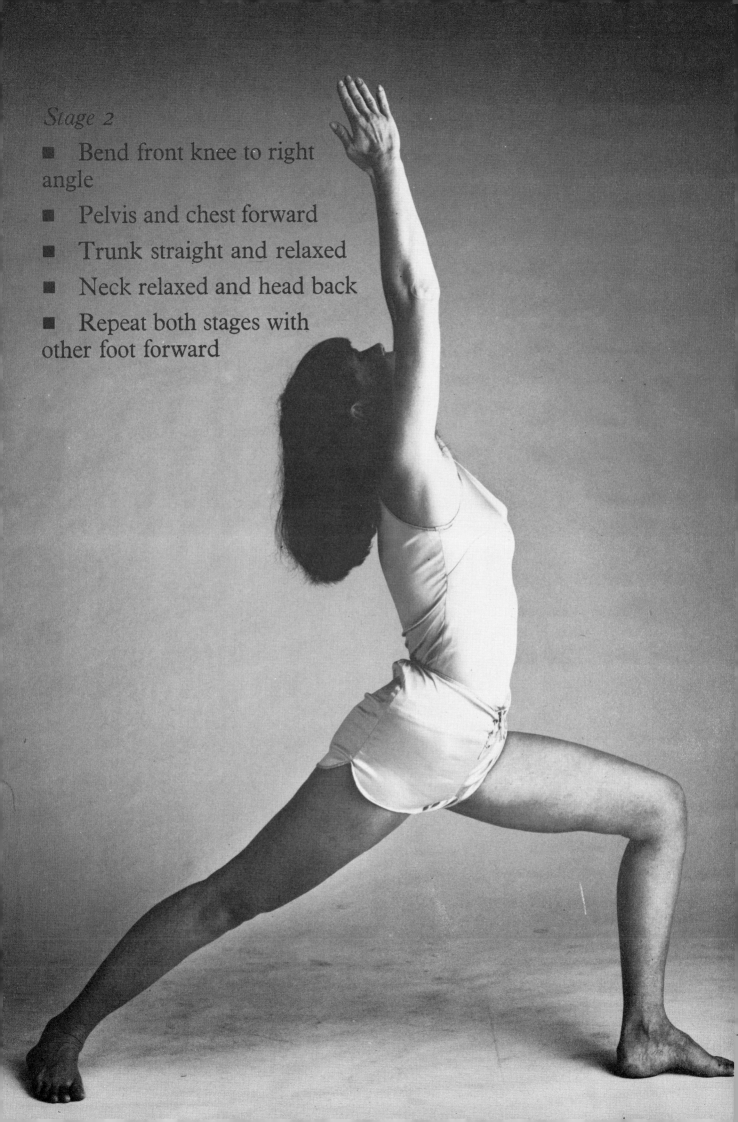

Stage 2

- Bend front knee to right angle
- Pelvis and chest forward
- Trunk straight and relaxed
- Neck relaxed and head back
- Repeat both stages with other foot forward

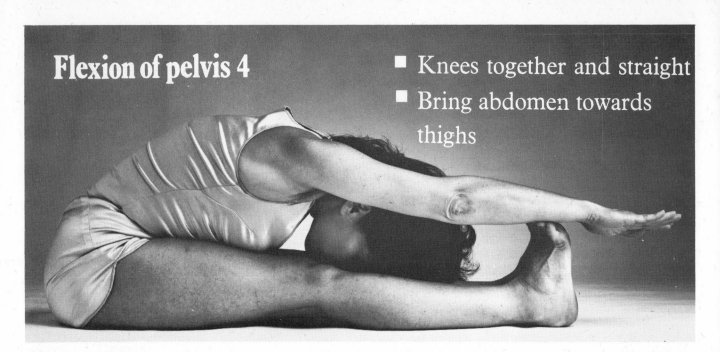

Flexion of pelvis 4

- Knees together and straight
- Bring abdomen towards thighs

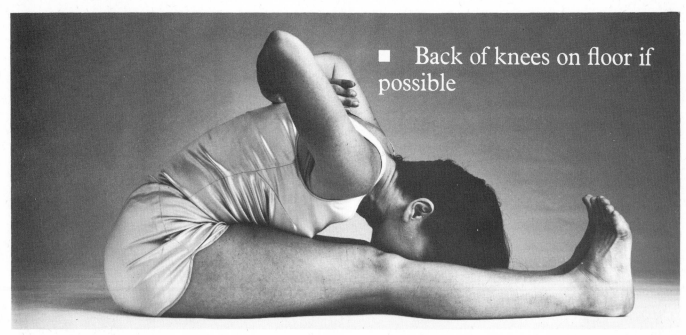

- Back of knees on floor if possible

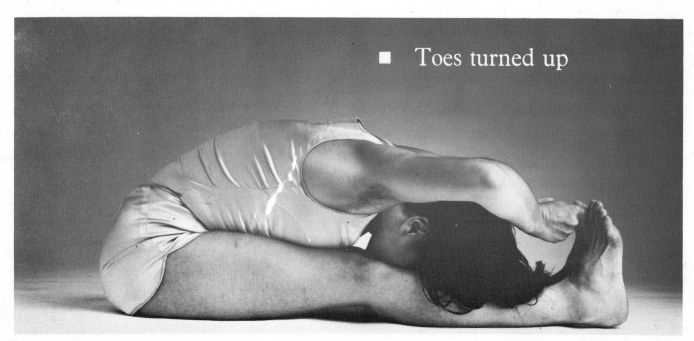

- Toes turned up

■ When first starting, try to lower elbows to floor and clasp ankles, then heels

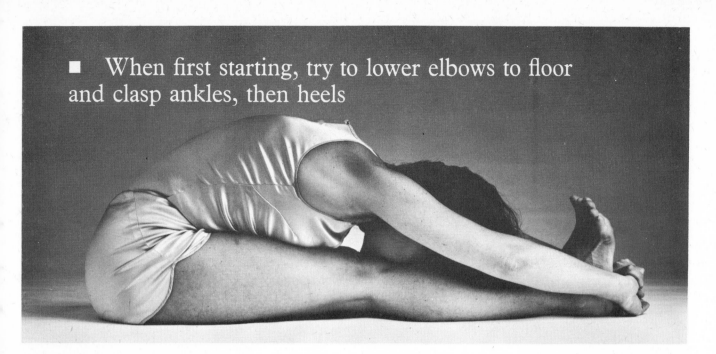

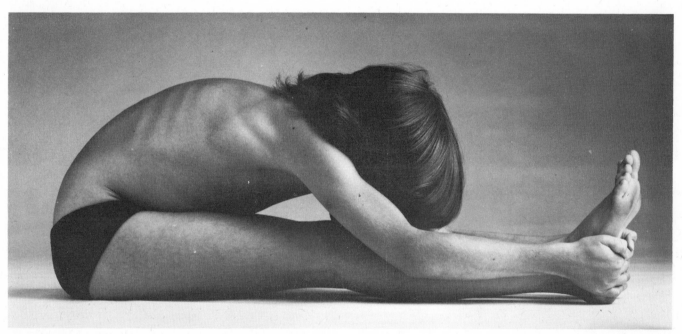

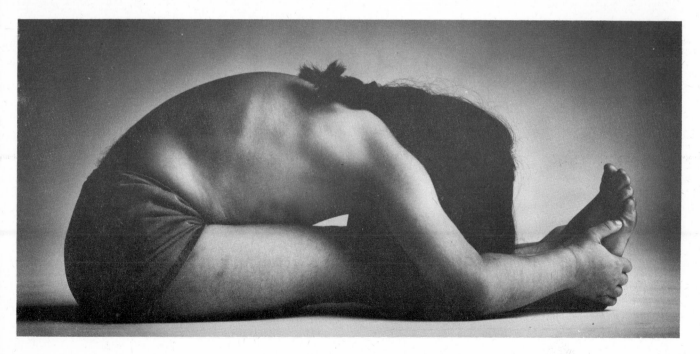

Flexion of pelvis 5

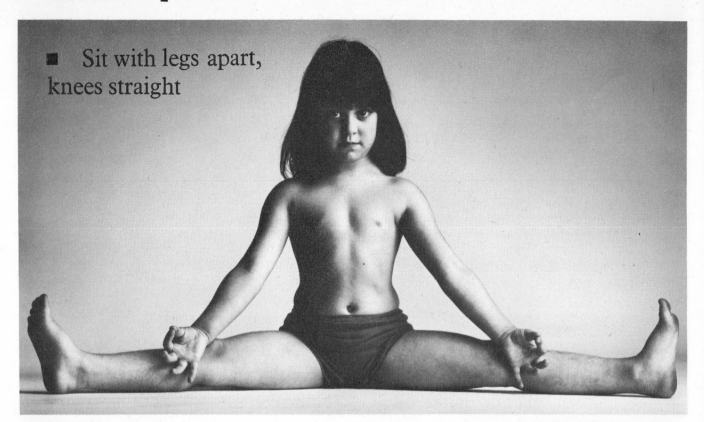

■ Sit with legs apart, knees straight

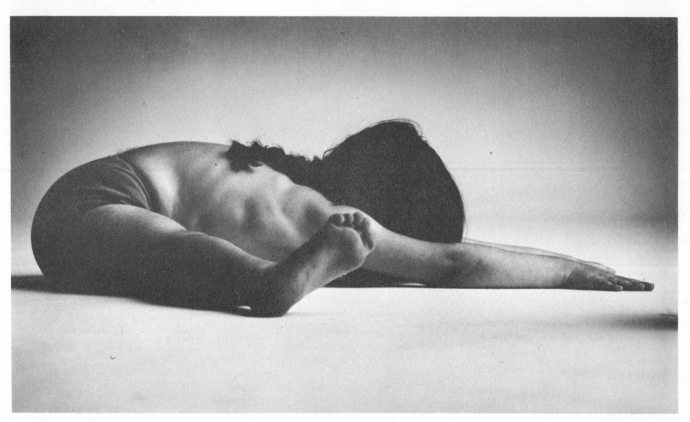

■ Reach forward and down

■ Aim to touch floor with chin, in order to keep spine as straight as possible

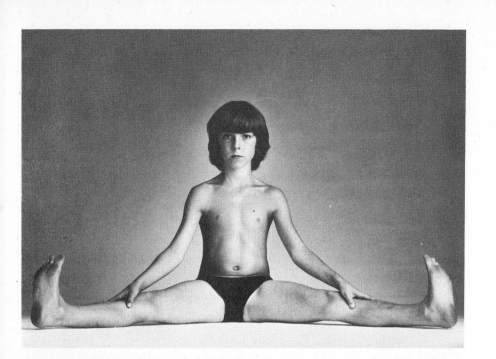

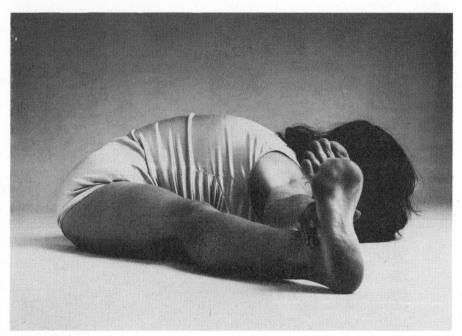

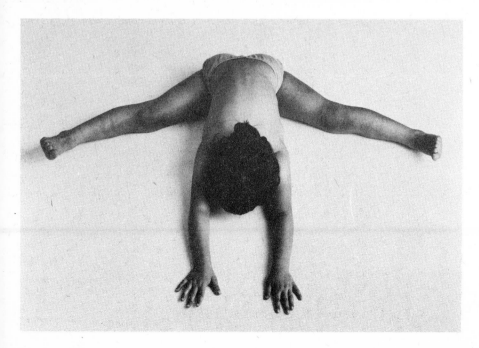

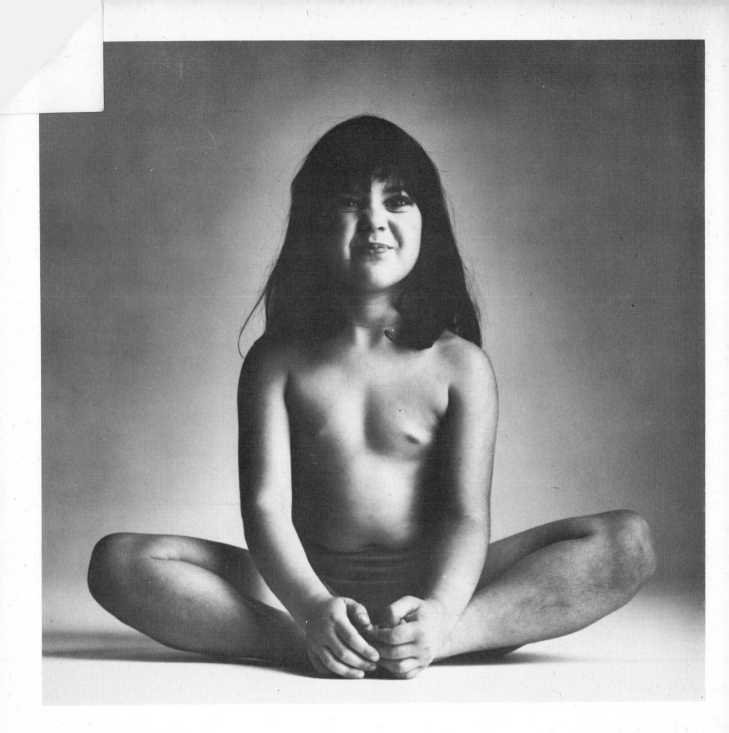

Flexion of pelvis 6

- Sit with knees out and bent

- Soles of feet together

- Draw feet towards groin

- Trunk straight and relaxed

- Clasping toes press knees down towards floor

(Only when the above is easy, try reaching forward and down to place head on floor)

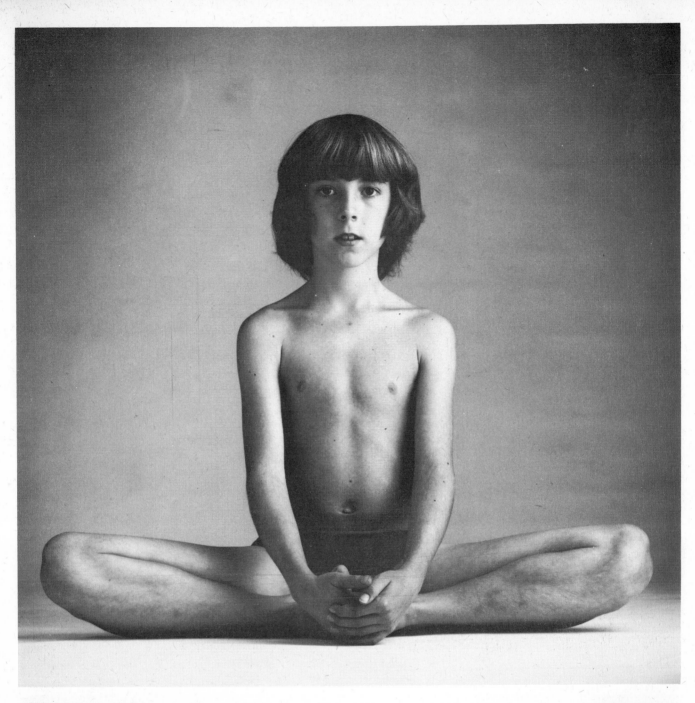

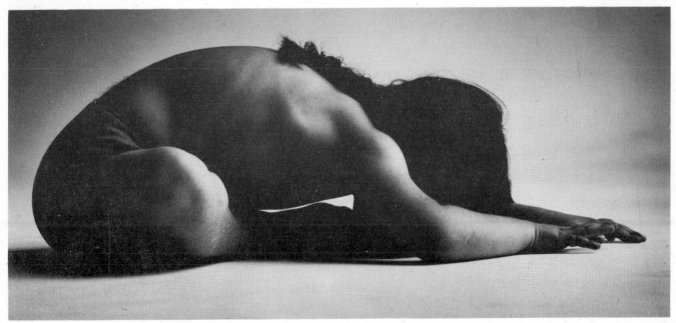

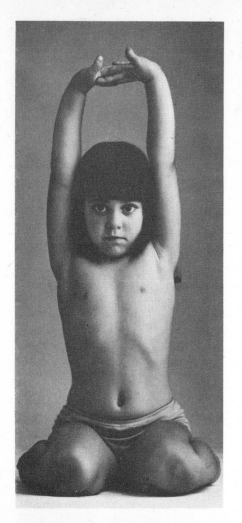
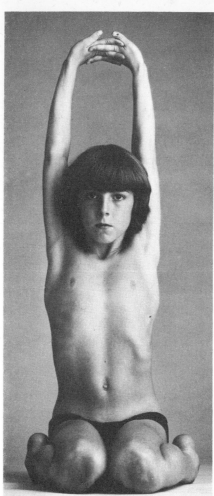

Flexion of pelvis 7

Stage 1

- Sit between feet knees together
- Stretch arms above head interlacing fingers
- Palms to ceiling
- Shoulders down
- Buttocks in contact with floor

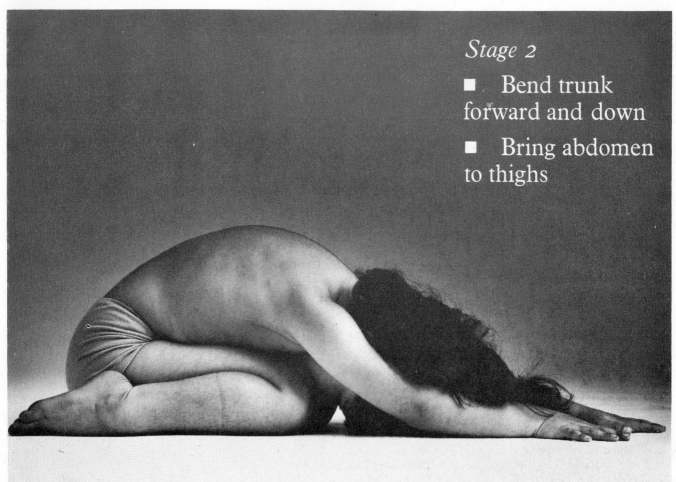

Stage 2

- Bend trunk forward and down
- Bring abdomen to thighs

Extension of pelvis, spine and shoulders

Stage 1

■ As previous Stage 1

■ Lean back on elbows

Stage 2

■ Ease yourself to lying position between feet

■ Bring hands easily over head

■ Keep knees together

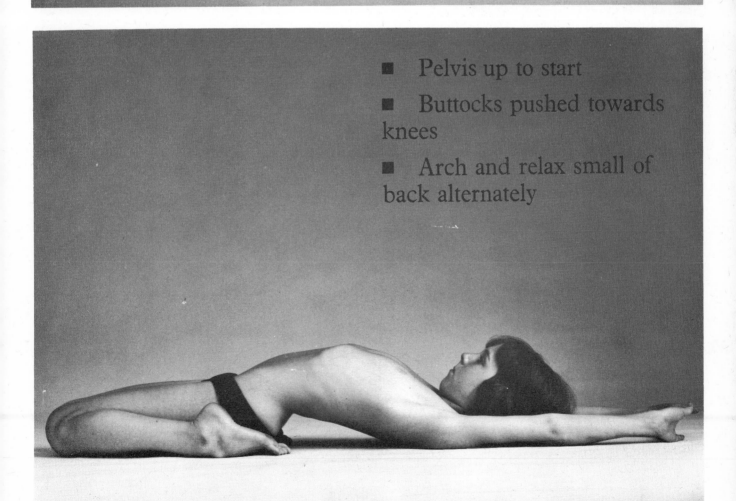

■ Pelvis up to start

■ Buttocks pushed towards knees

■ Arch and relax small of back alternately

...ension of pelvis, spine and shoulders

- Kneel with knees together and feet slightly apart

- Bend spine backward, hands on heels

- Push pelvis forward until thighs are vertical

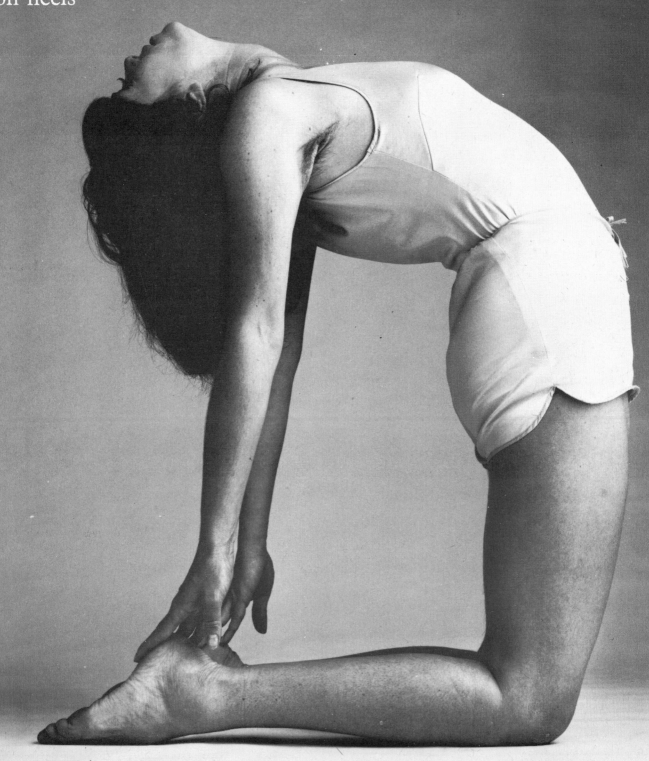

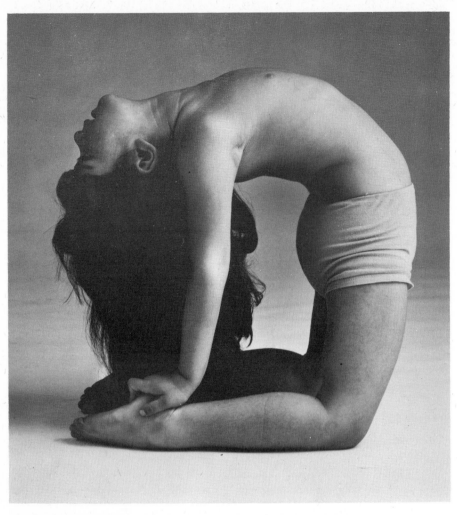

When more advanced

- Hands on ankles
- Arms straight
- Trunk parallel to floor, making a square

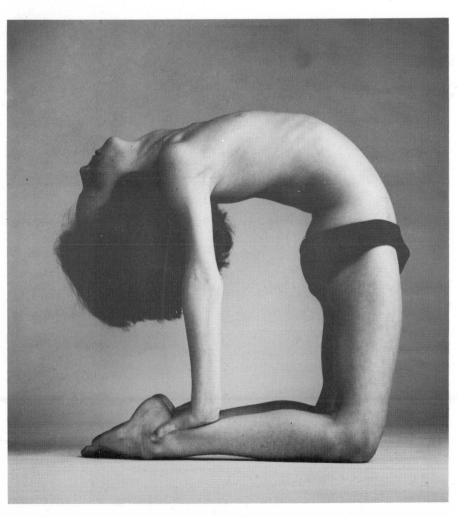

Extension of spine, pelvis, knees and ankles

- Lie face down on floor
- Place hands near shoulders
- Push curving spine backwards
- Keep shoulders down
- Chest forward

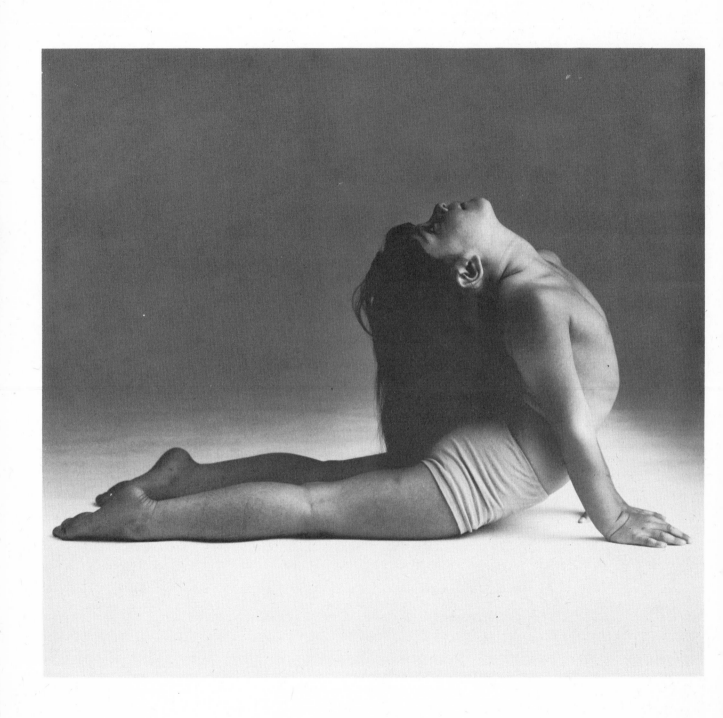

Extension of spine, variation

- Progress to balance on insteps and arms

- Face parallel to ceiling

- Back of neck relaxed

- Start with legs in contact with floor

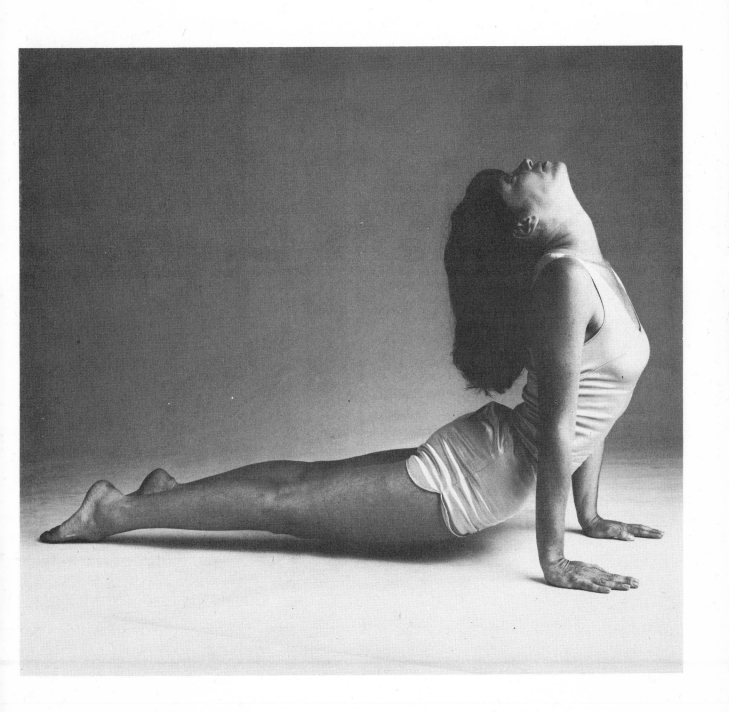

Extension of spine, bending back fully

- Start by lying on floor
- Palms by ears
- Fingers towards feet
- Keep feet slightly apart, bend knees and draw feet in close to buttocks
- Raise trunk and rest crown of head on floor

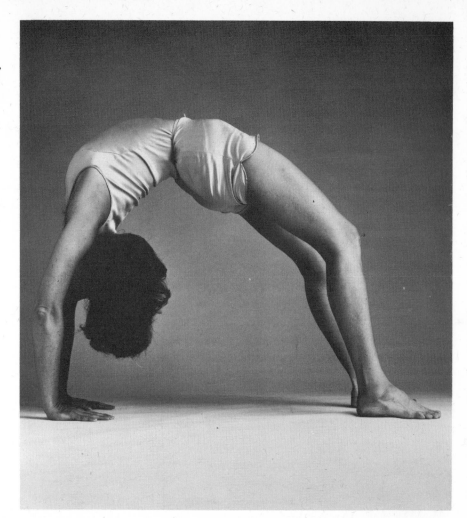

- Lift trunk and head, arching back fully
- Weight on palms and soles of feet

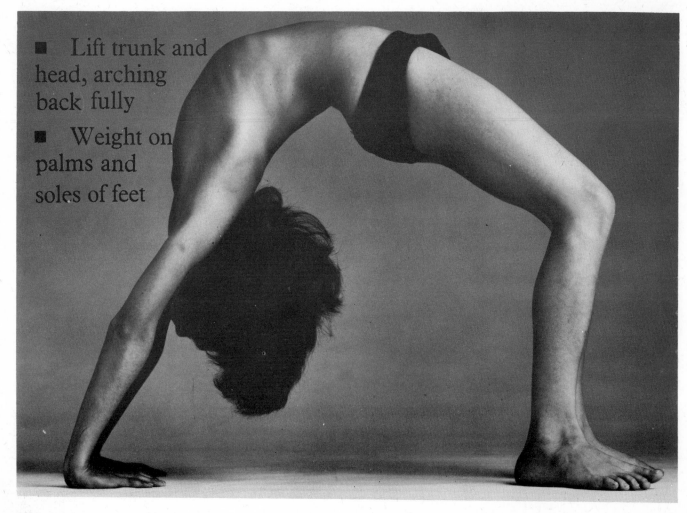

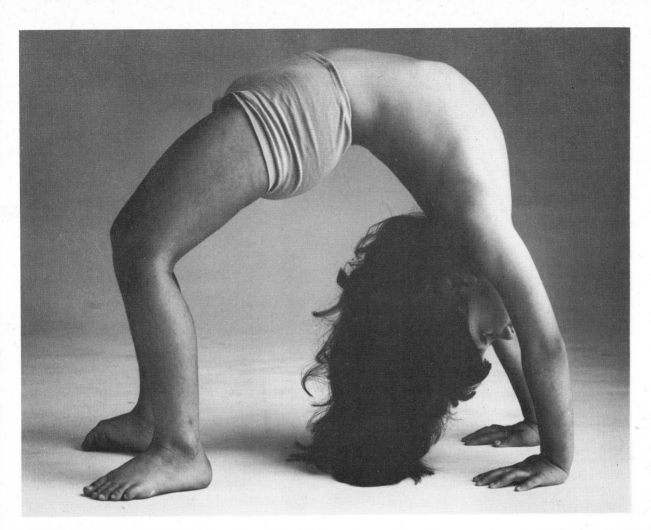

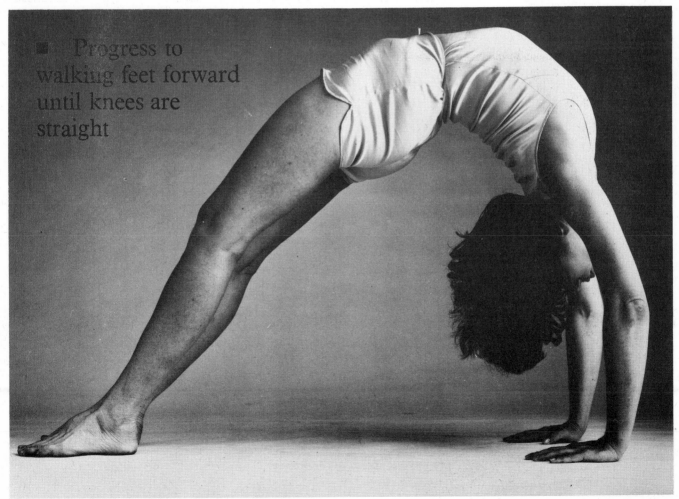

■ Progress to
walking feet forward
until knees are
straight

Strengthening abdominal muscles

- Sit with knees straight and together
- Lean back, raising straight legs above level of head

- Arms parallel to floor
- Spine as straight as possible

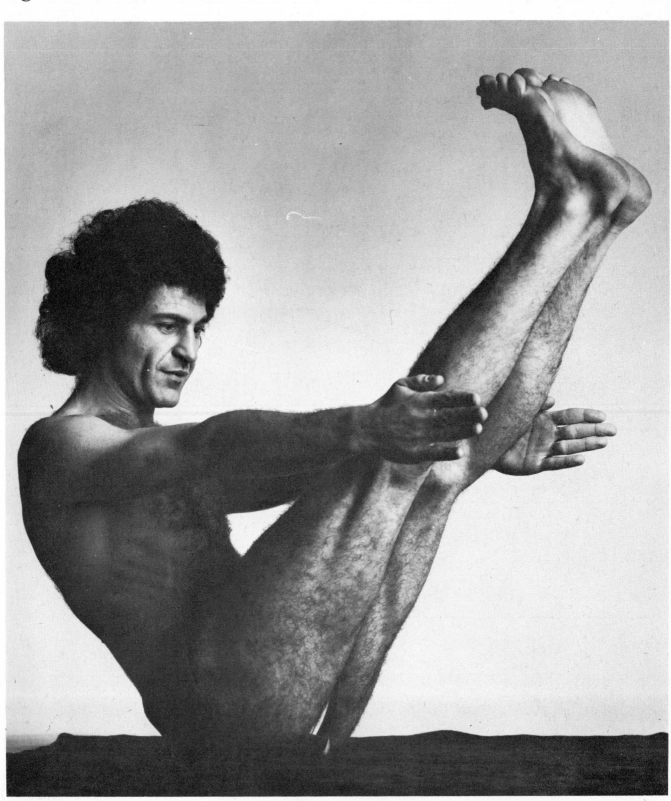

Spinal twist

- Sit with knees straight and feet together

- Bring one foot over opposite thigh and place flat on floor

- Bend other knee, and slide foot next to buttock

- Turn trunk towards foot by buttock, twisting spine as much as possible, especially between shoulders

- Extend arm over outside upright knee

- Arm straight and hand gripping foot

- Other hand resting on floor, head looking over shoulder

- Shoulders open and level

- Repeat for opposite side

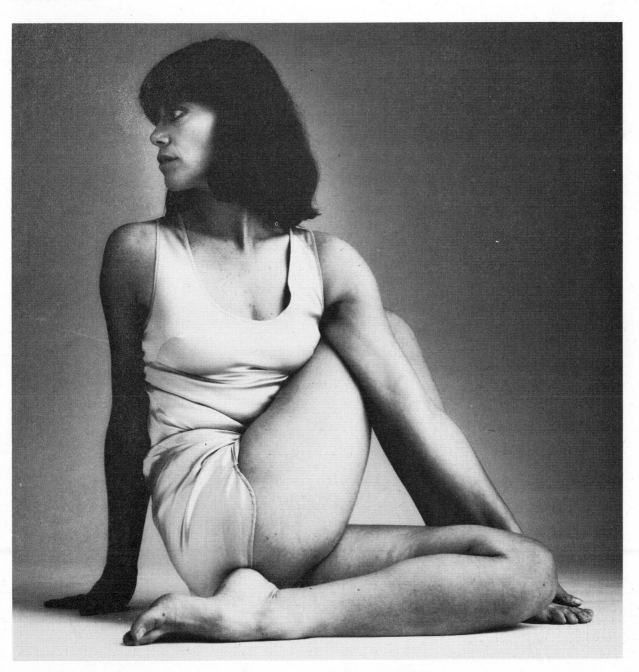

Head balance

- Use wall to start for security, and folded blanket for head and elbow comfort

- Kneel with linked hands together on floor

- Elbows apart at shoulder width

- Head cupped by hands

- Crown of head on floor, back of neck straight

- Transfer weight on to feet

- Walk in until thighs touch chest

- Transfer weight to head and arms

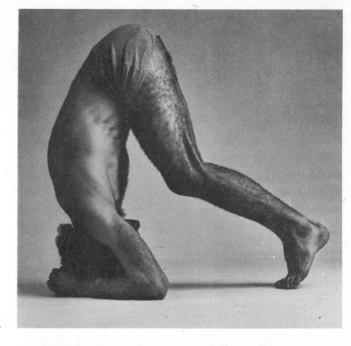

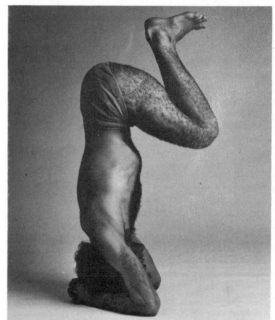

- Unfold until knees point at ceiling

- Straighten legs

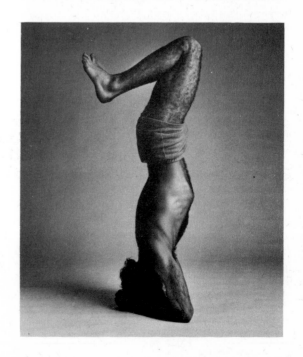

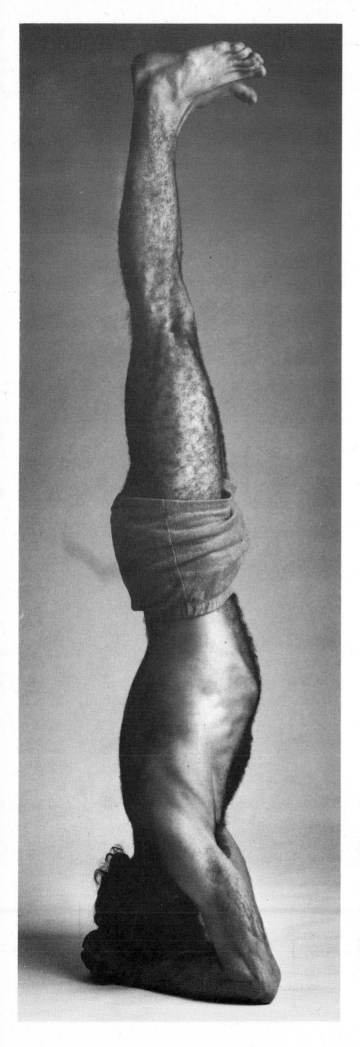

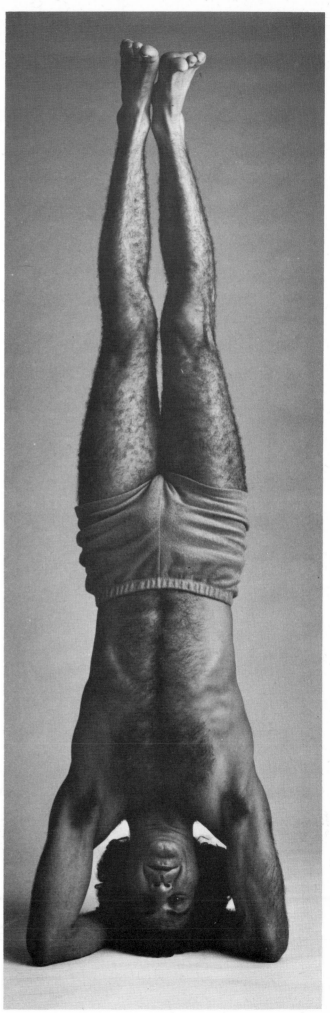

Head balance

In posture checks

- Shoulder blades lifting up towards hips
- Armpits forward
- Buttocks upward to heels
- Pelvis level
- Try to avoid arching back
- Stretch back of legs more than front
- Knees inwards to each other
- Feet easy

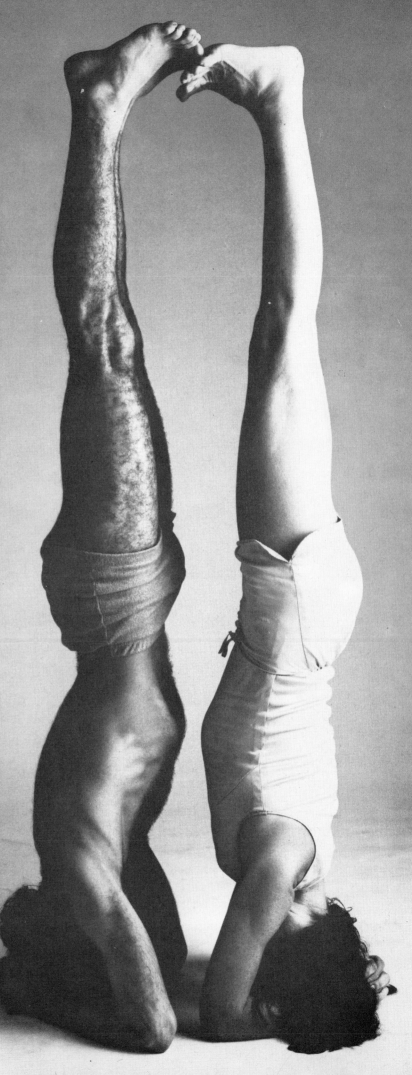

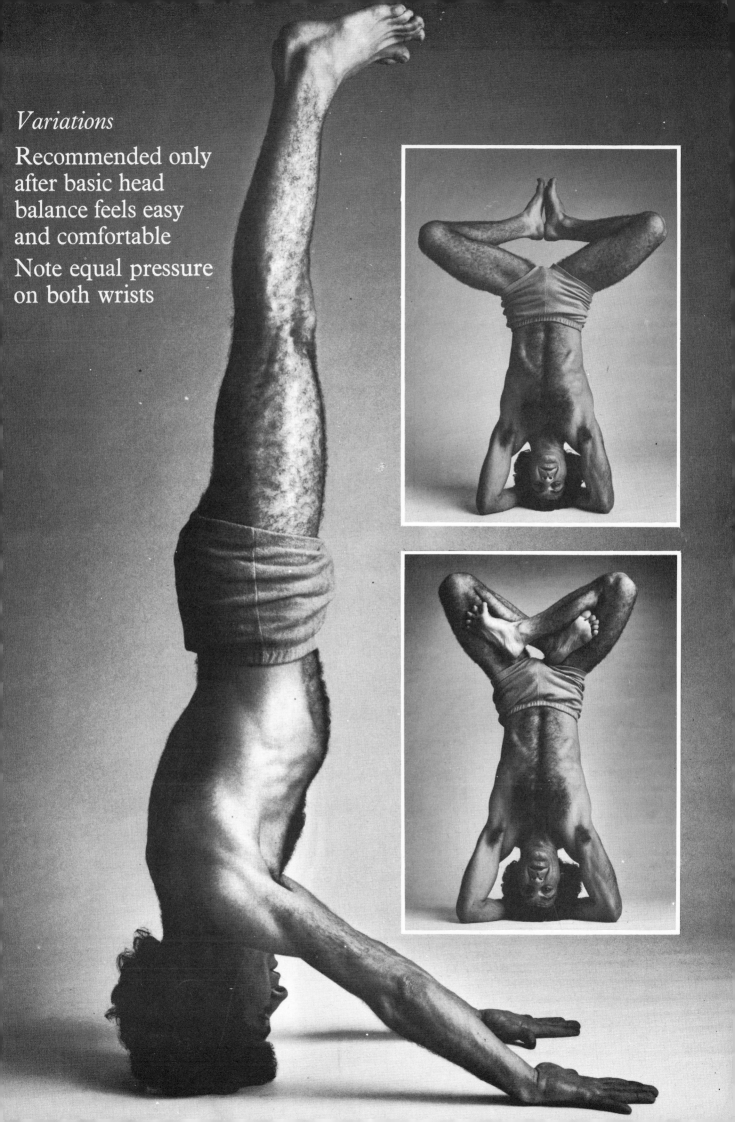

Variations

Recommended only
after basic head
balance feels easy
and comfortable

Note equal pressure
on both wrists

Shoulder balance

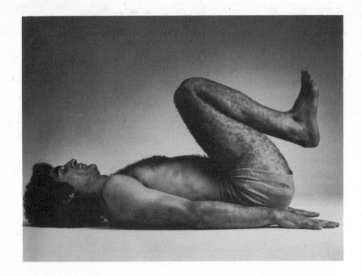

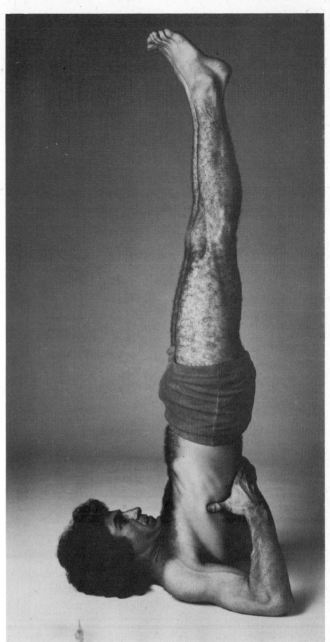

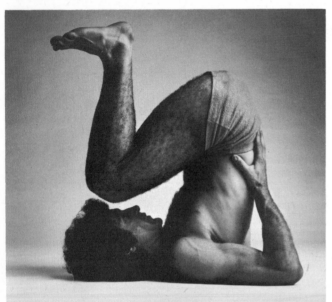

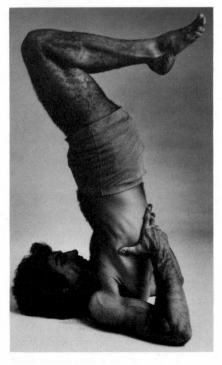

- Lie flat on back
- Chin tucked in
- Palms on floor
- Swing knees to forehead
- Hands on small of back
- Slide hands towards floor for extra support
- Point knees towards ceiling
- Straighten legs

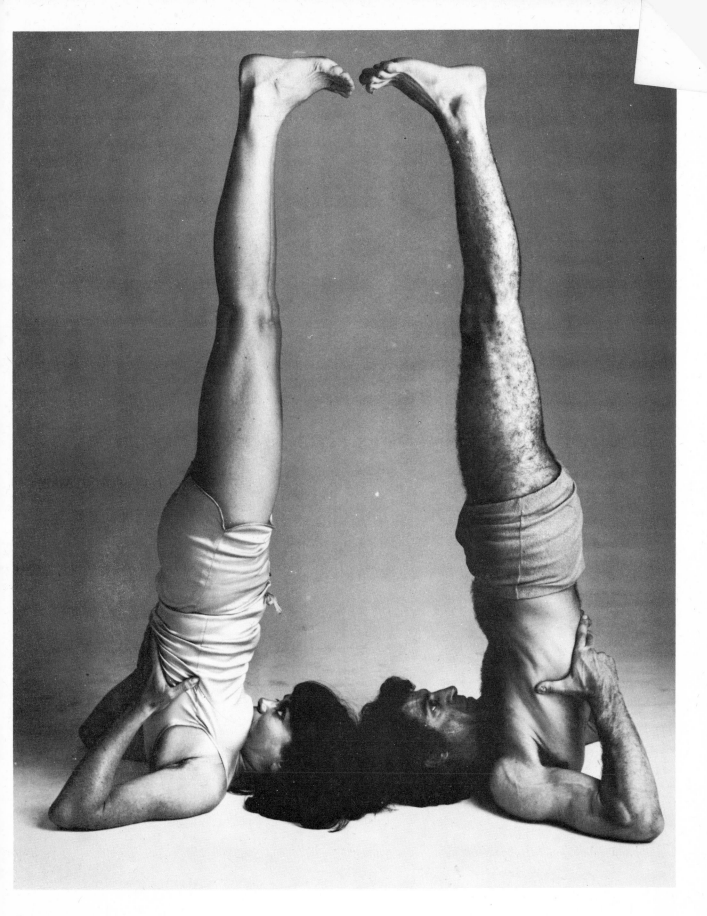

In posture checks

■ Lift trunk upwards and as perpendicular to the floor as possible

■ Knees straight and facing slightly inward

■ Feet relaxed

Full back stretch

The plough

- Basic posture as for Shoulder Balance

- Legs straight over head using hands to support back

- Push gently to let legs rest on floor

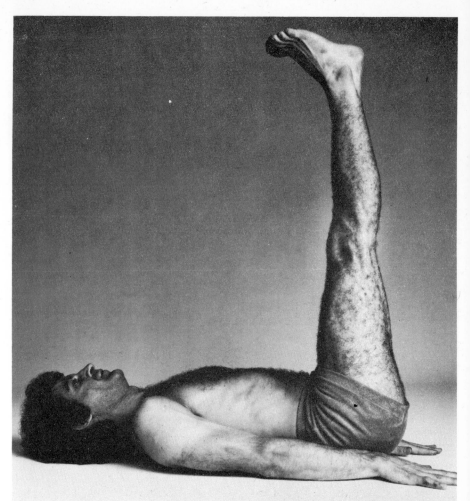

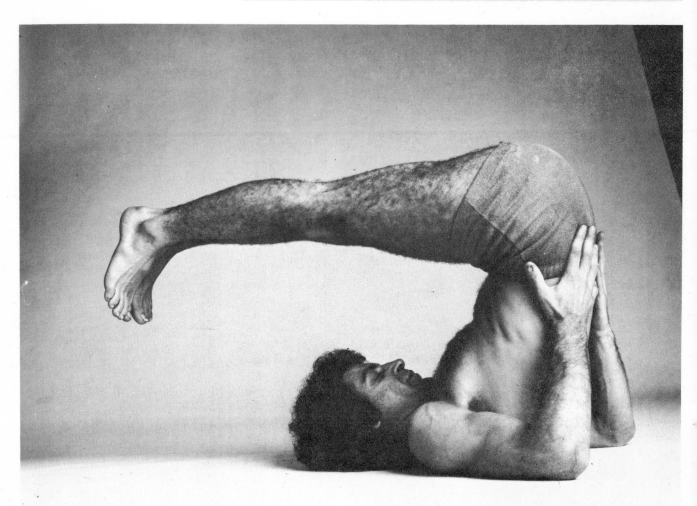

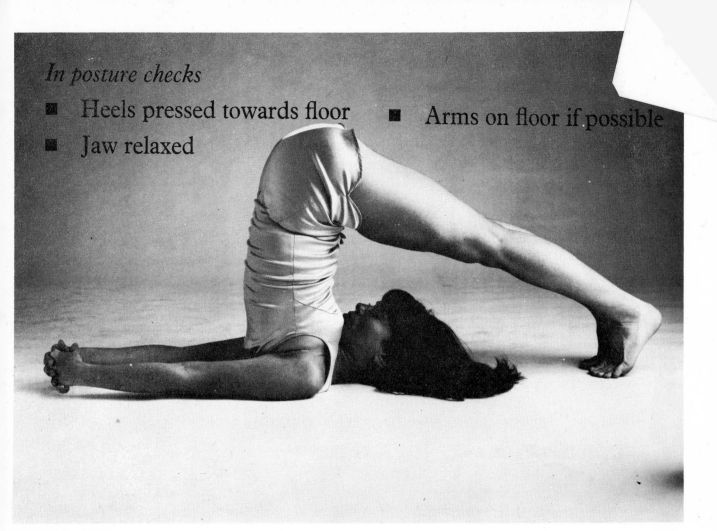

In posture checks
- Heels pressed towards floor
- Jaw relaxed
- Arms on floor if possible

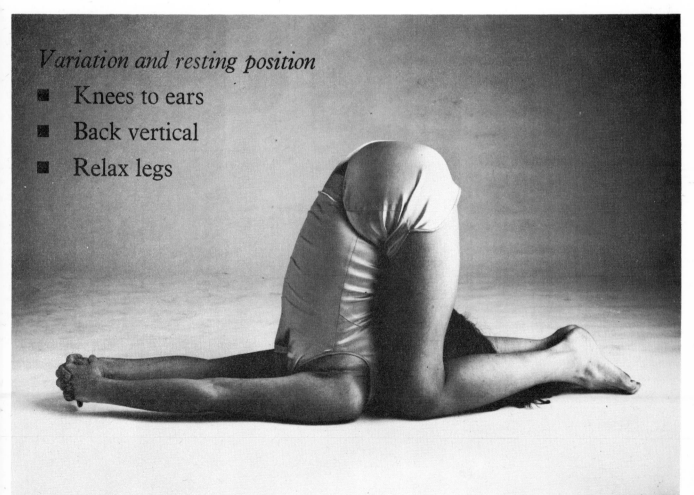

Variation and resting position
- Knees to ears
- Back vertical
- Relax legs

or hands

Our hands are simple-looking yet ingenious structures. They are the basis of all our technical progress: the first tool of the intellect.

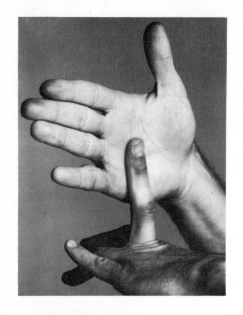

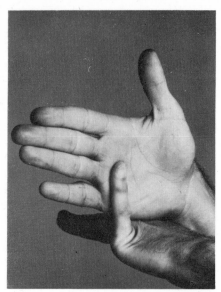

■ Each finger can be bent at three different joints

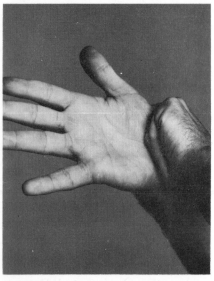

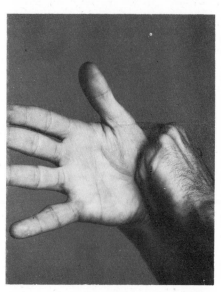

■ Press back each whole finger until it is at near right angles to its palm

■ Flex the middle joint of each finger fully. The joints may make a cracking sound. Do not worry!

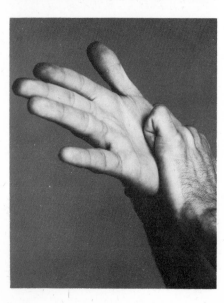

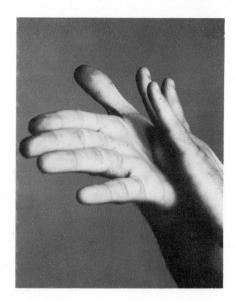

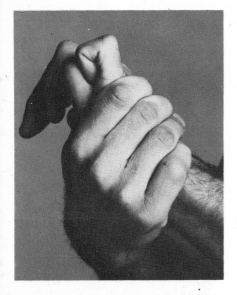

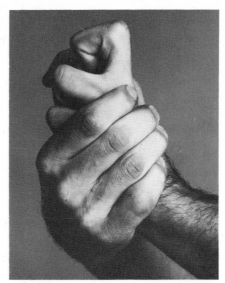

■ Flex the top finger joint as much as possible

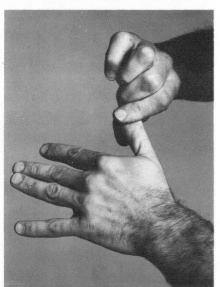

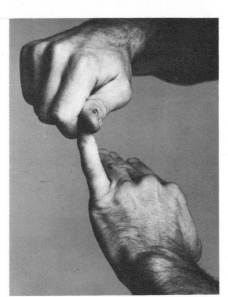

■ Rotate each finger and thumb first one way then the other

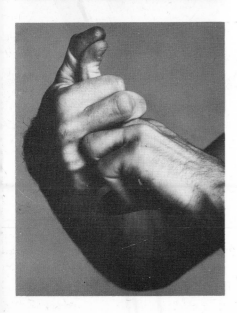

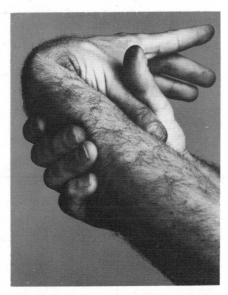

■ Each top finger joint may be bent backwards

■ Bend the wrist and press thumb down towards lower arm

■ Finally shake both hands as freely as possible

To some the nature of our body is shown by its freedom of movement and its balanced uprightness.

Mechanically we have the capacity for a large variety of movements, made possible by engineering design of a high order. But we seem to lack a proper understanding of the natural structure, function and possible range of our body movements. They require conscious effort to begin with but, like learning to ride a bicycle, after a while the more unconscious and reflex they become, the better.

Mechanically, physiologically and psychologically, it appears we are all compelled to struggle for a state of balance or equilibrium. Our body, like all other objects on earth, is continuously subject to the pull of gravity, and saving of weight is mechanically very desirable, since it saves fuel, minimizes wear and tear and improves efficiency. There are only three ways in which weight may be supported, and we support weight in all three ways. It may sit—our head sits upon our spine. It may hang—our arms hang from our shoulder-girdle. It may be braced—our hip bones brace our sacrum at the base of our spine. Saving of weight and achieving better balance depends a great deal on our knowledge and familiarity of where and how our body weights sit, hang or are braced, and on the degree to which we can realize the meaning and sense of balance.

The ball and socket joints of our pelvis and shoulders, while having a great deal of movement in all directions, are also under most stress and strain. We know many of us cannot touch our toes while our knees are straight because of tight hamstring muscles, but that tight pectoral muscles restrict the degree through which our arms may be raised is not always appreciated.

Nearly all the movement positions and balancings in this series concentrate to some degree or other on these two areas, and practising them seems to increase flexion, extension and rotation of most of our joints, and to promote a better curvature of our spine. In short, these practices are for those not satisfied with restricted body movements and an unnecessary body resistance to the pull of the earth's gravity.

We are told that Shiva is the Hindu God of Yoga and also the God of Dance. A psychiatrist friend of mine suggests that the yoga postures or 'asanas' seem to be static positions from the continuous movements of the Dance of Shiva.

ARTHUR BALASKAS

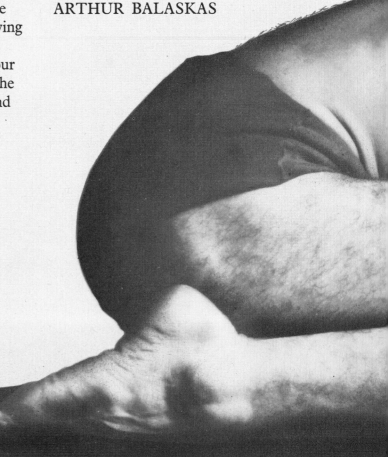

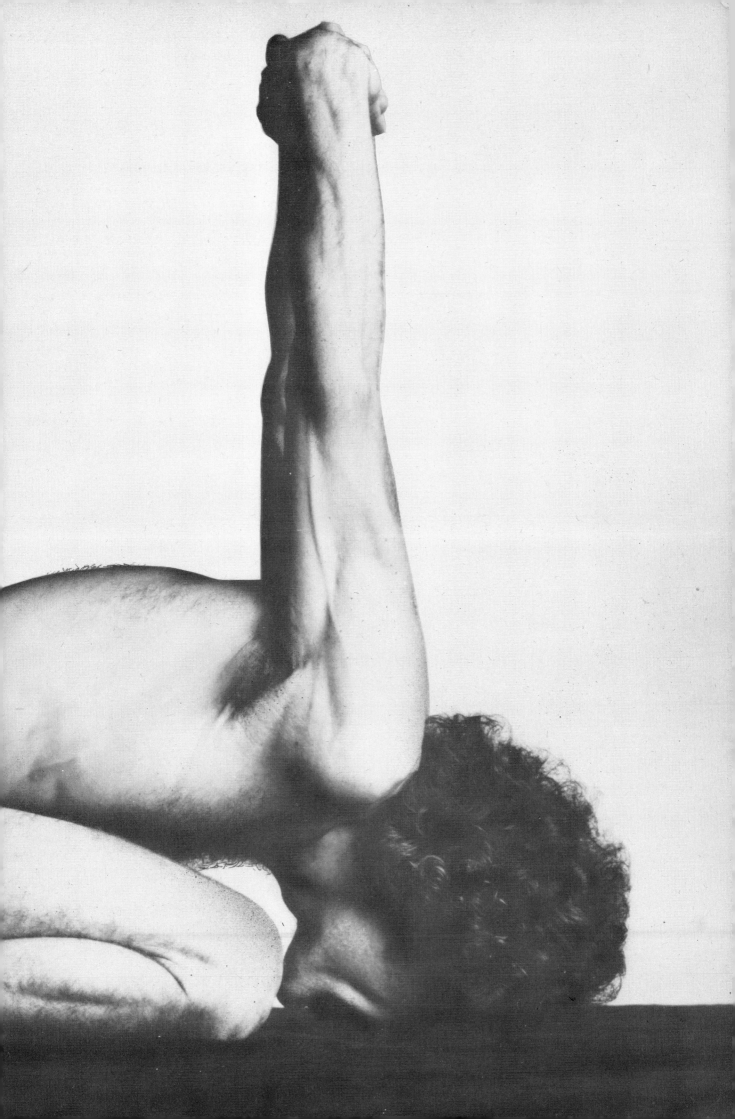

Notes and observations